Hooray! I Got a Cast Today!

Cast Care with Lyssy Loo

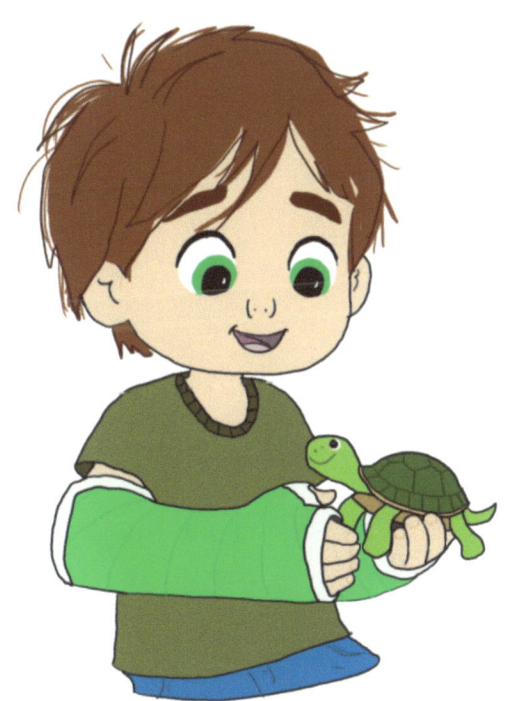

Written and illustrated by Alyssa Barré, MD.

ISBN: 9798883227522

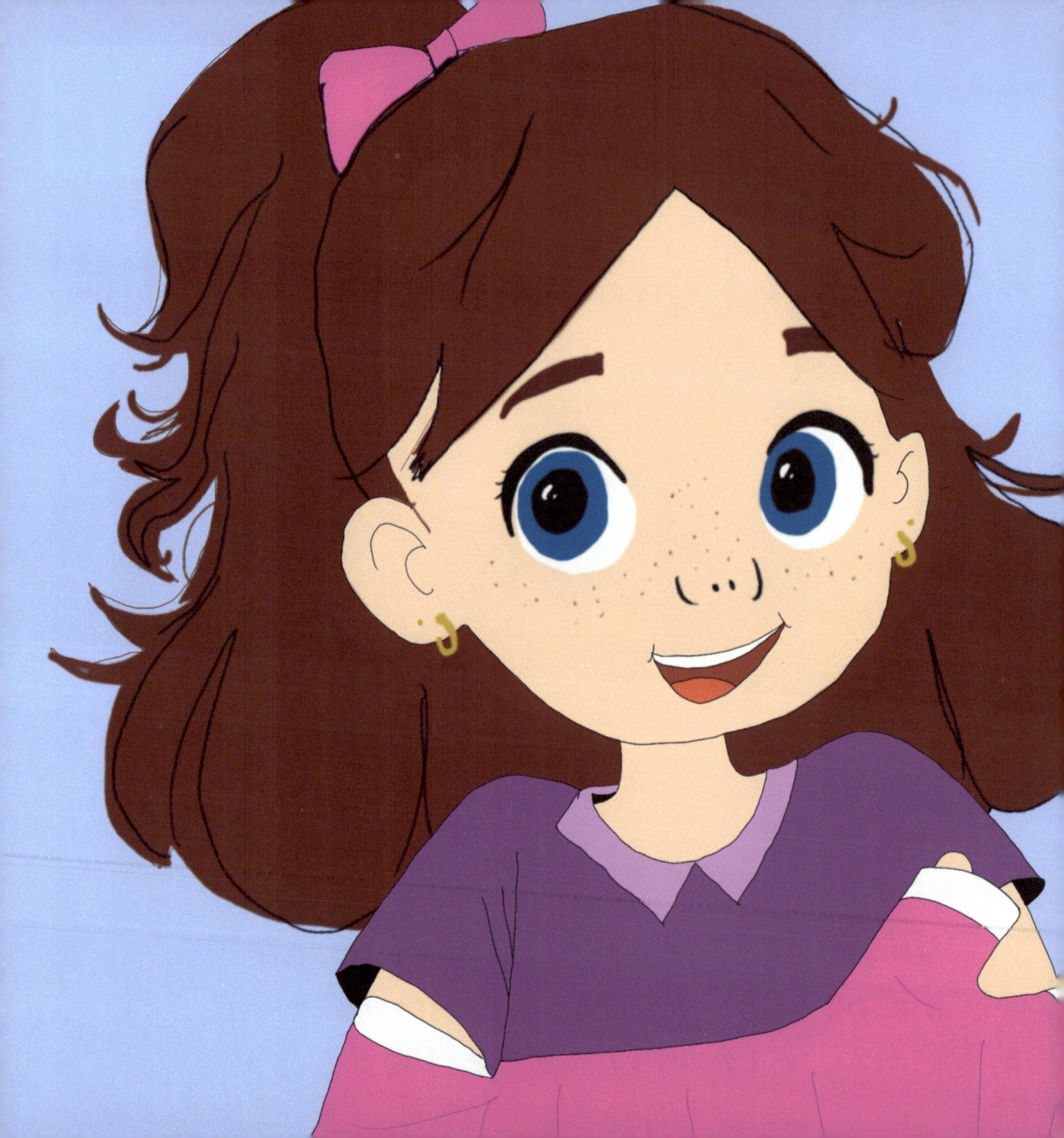

Hi there! My name is Lyssy Loo,
And I broke my arm, just like you!

A broken bone and a cast can seem
a little frightening,

But I will tell you all I know, and
you'll be back to playing fast as
lightning

Our bones are hard and strong.
They help us to run, and jump, and dance

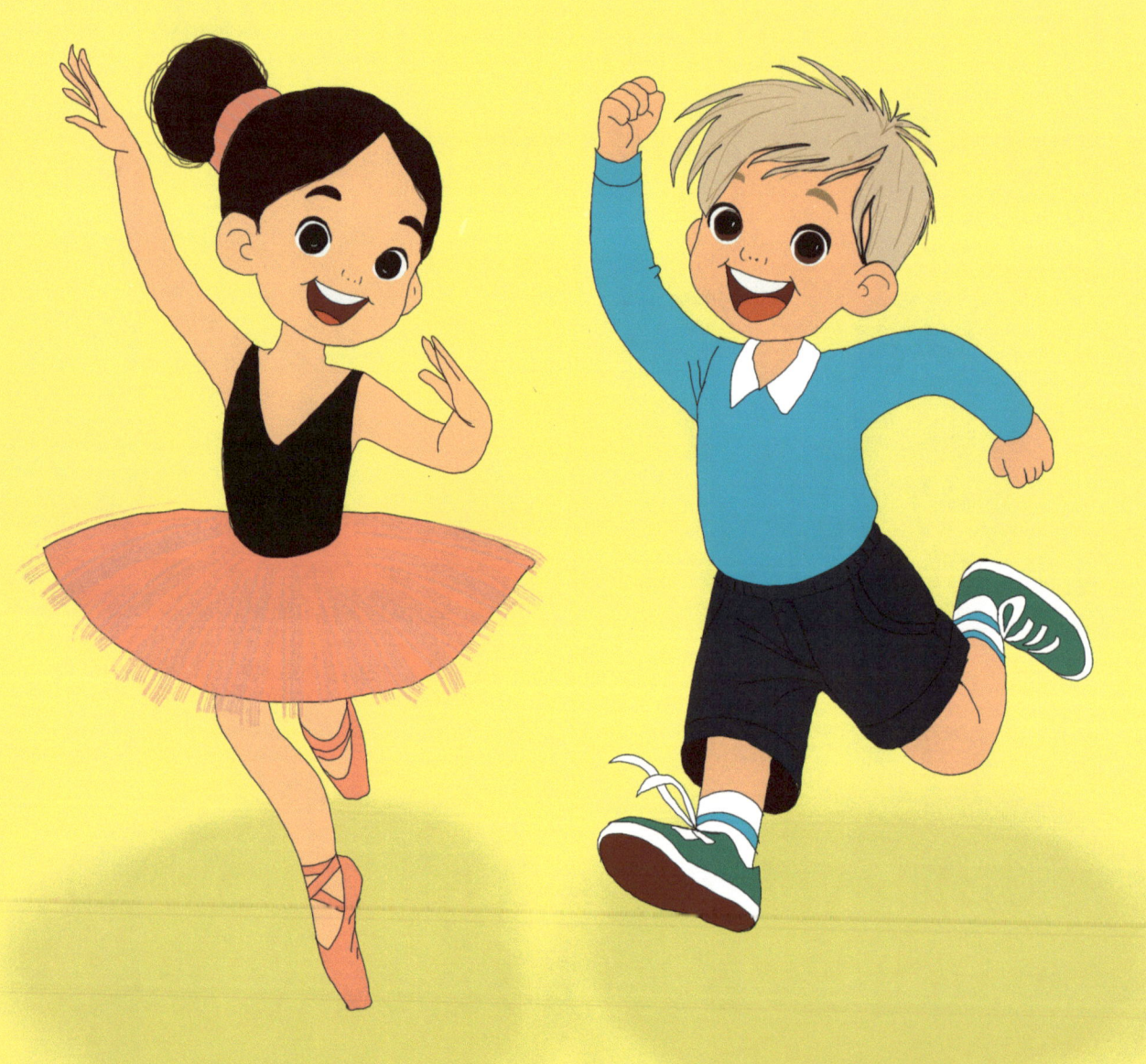

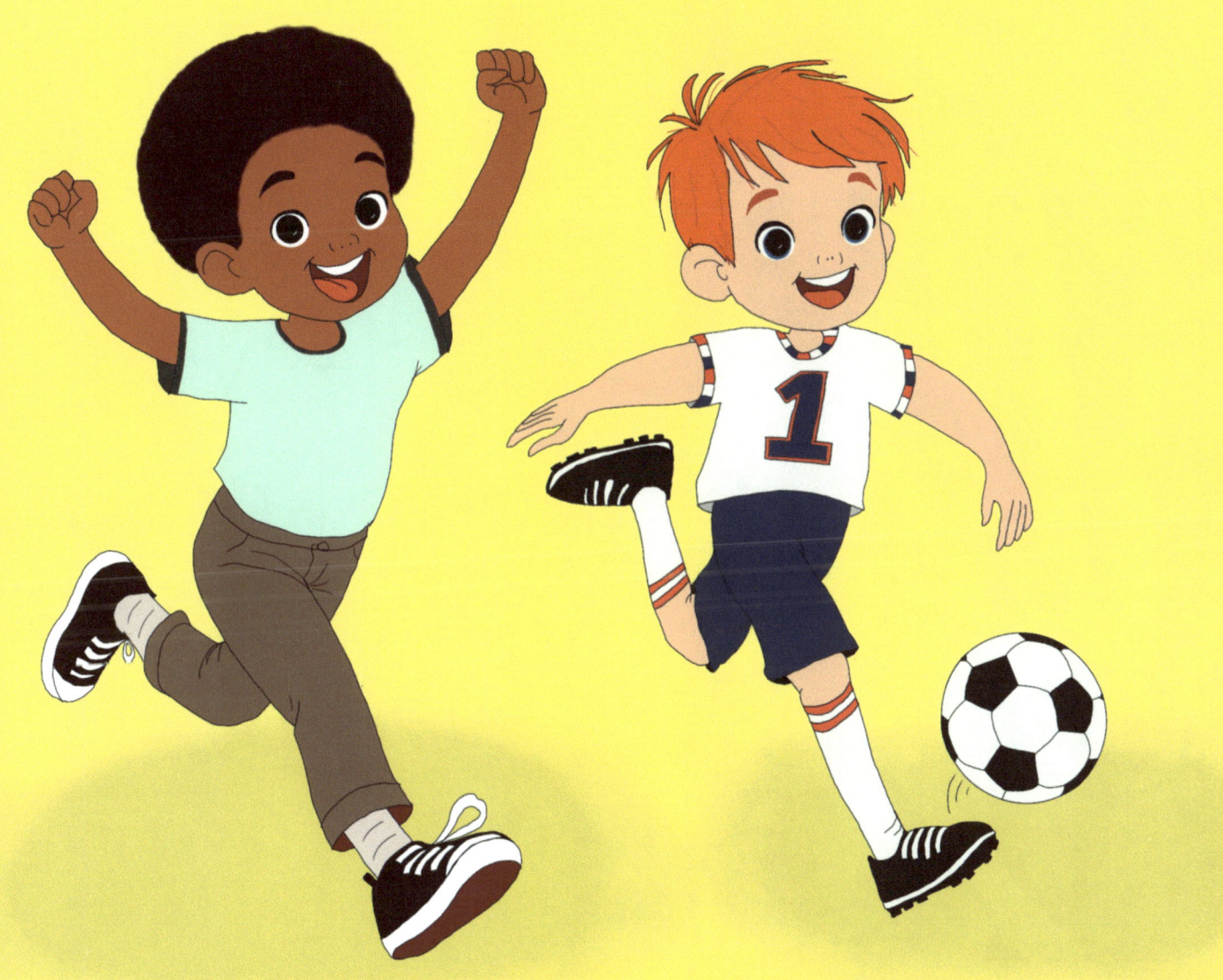

But if they break, they will need some time to heal,
And we must give them that chance

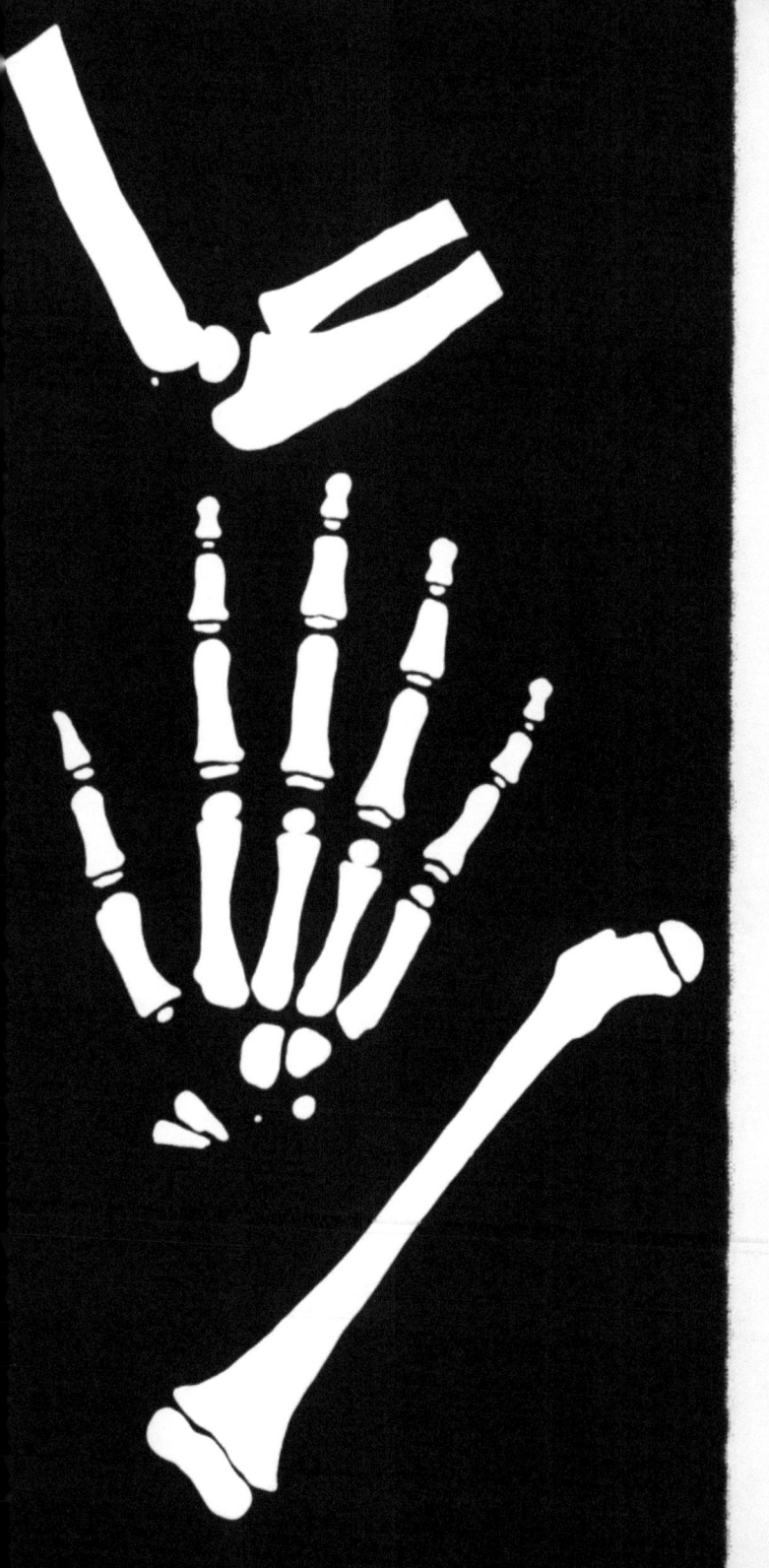

On the inside, your body knows just what to do

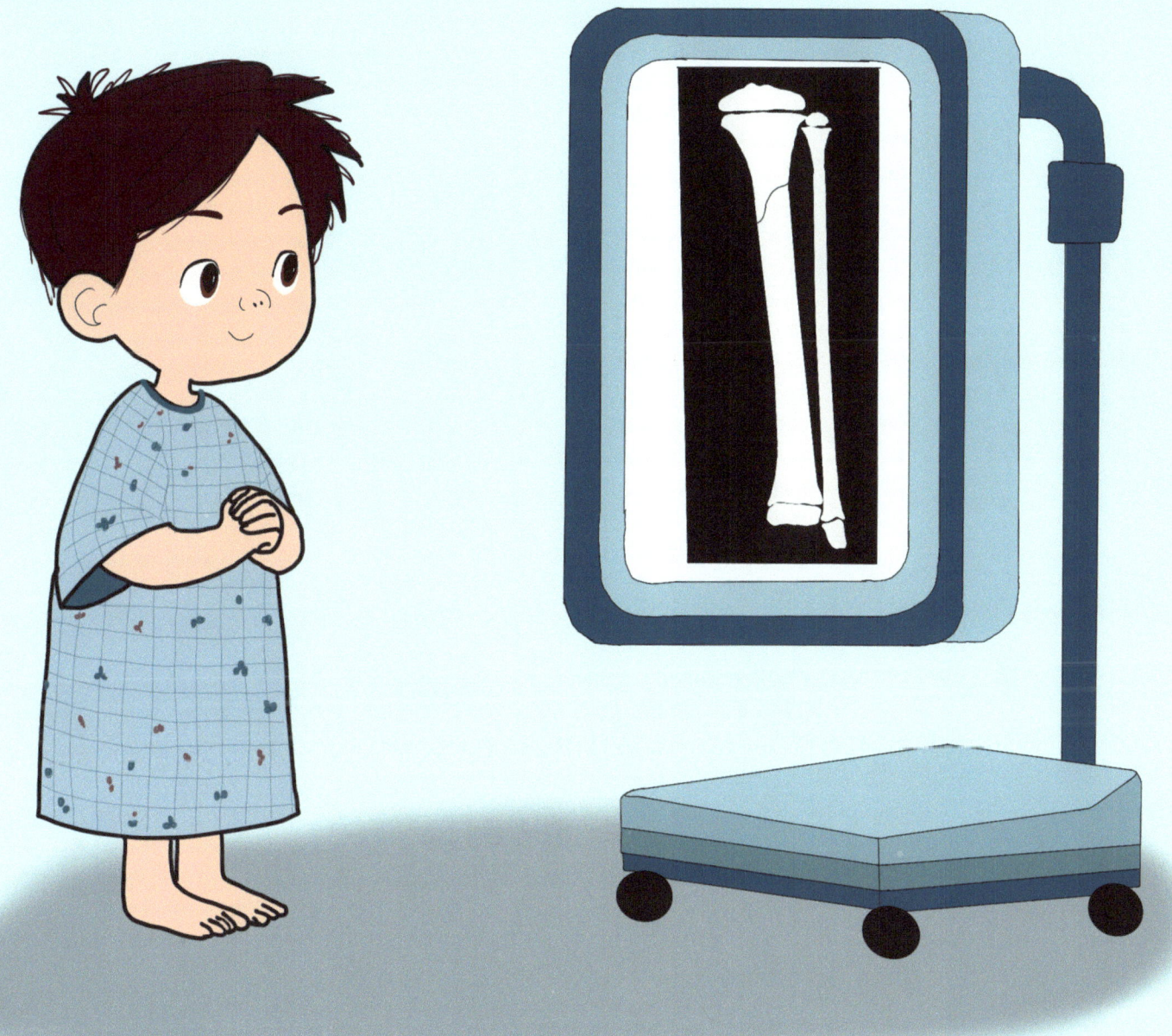

It's already busy working, filling in the gaps
to make your bone brand new

On the outside, a cast is like a turtle shell that's sturdy for protection

It keeps the bones safe inside while they undergo correction

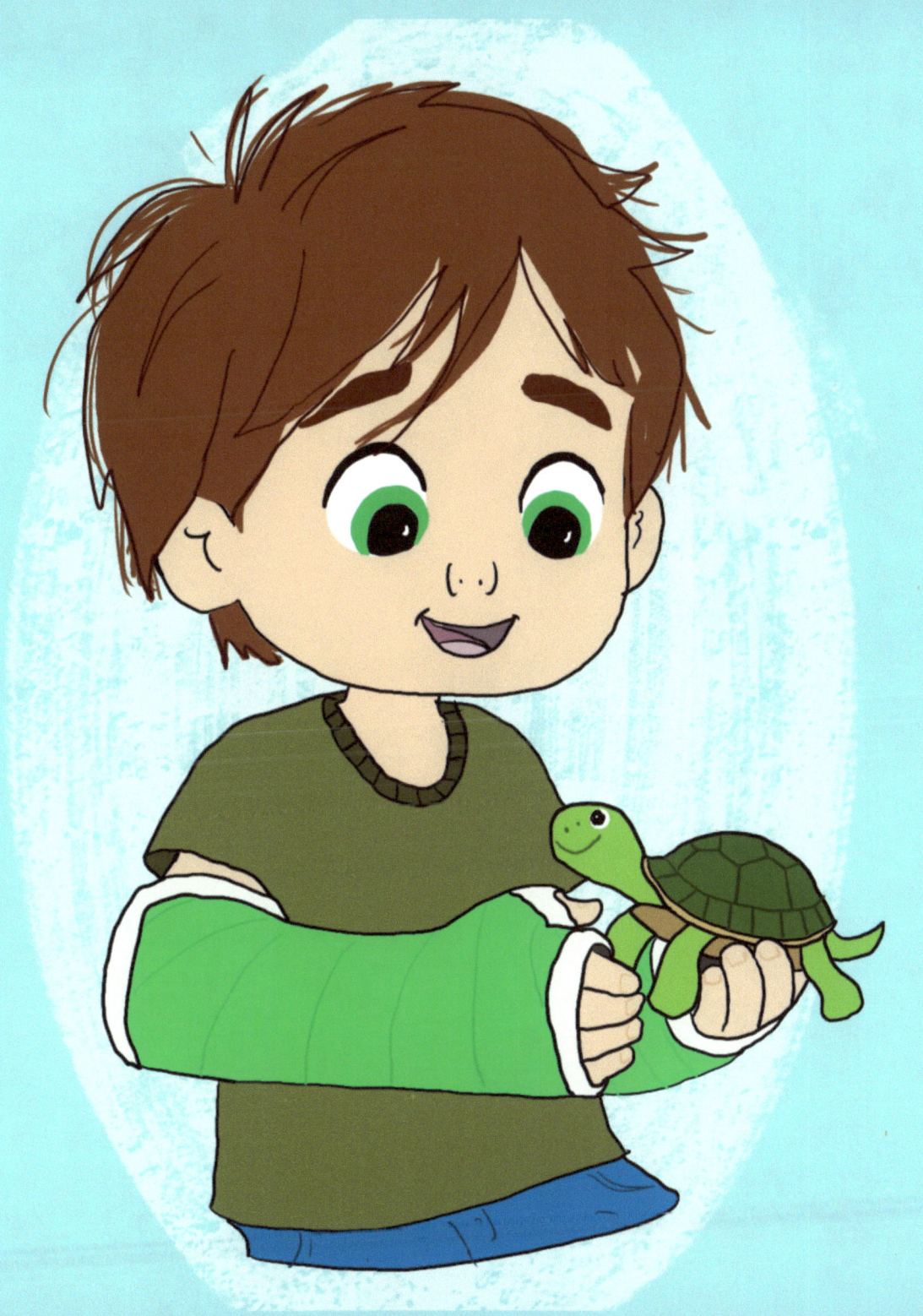

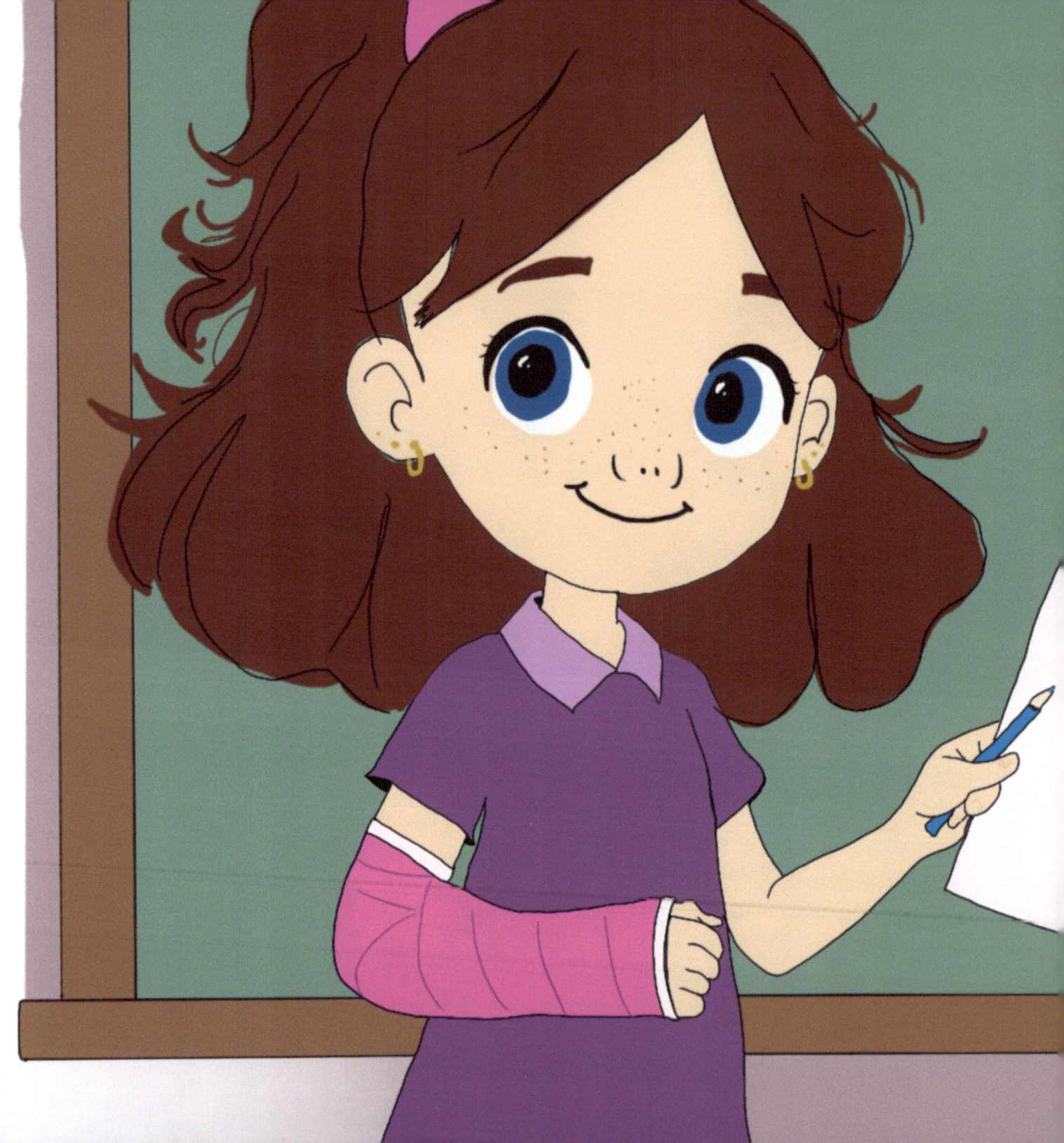

It takes a few weeks for the new bone to grow

And until that time, there are some rules that you must know

First, the cast will be ruined if it gets too wet

We must keep it covered in the bathtub, and no swimming just yet

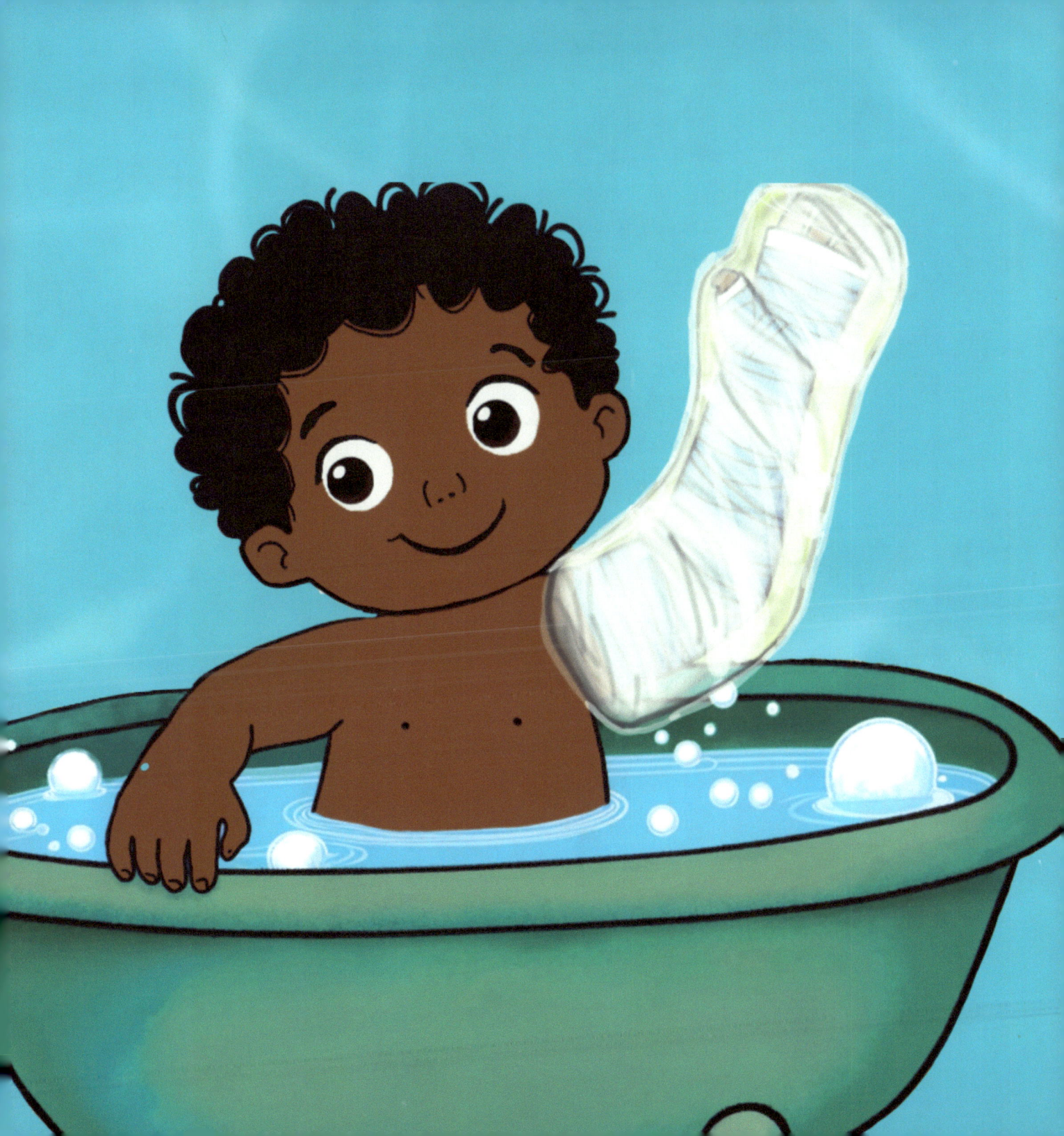

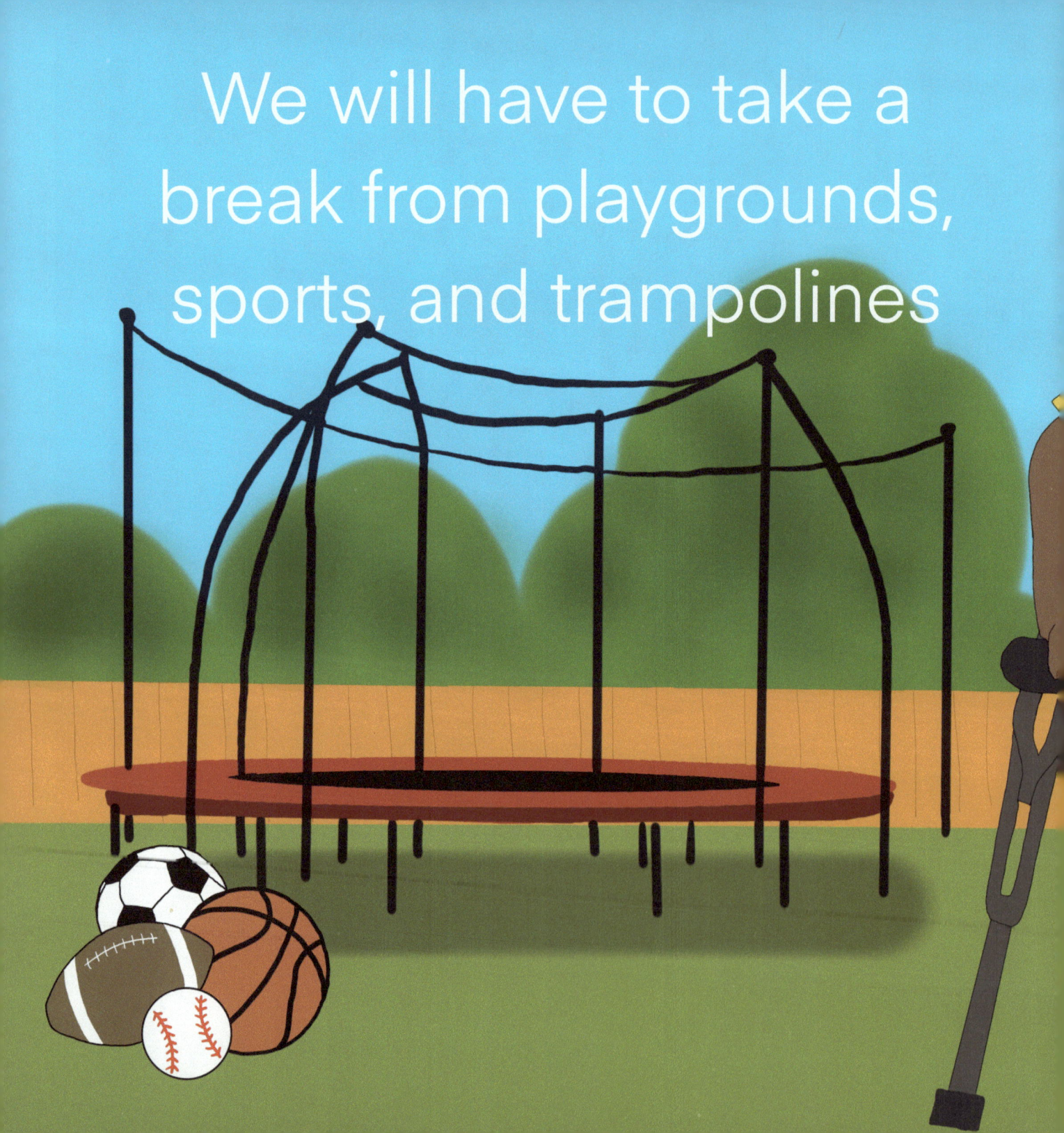

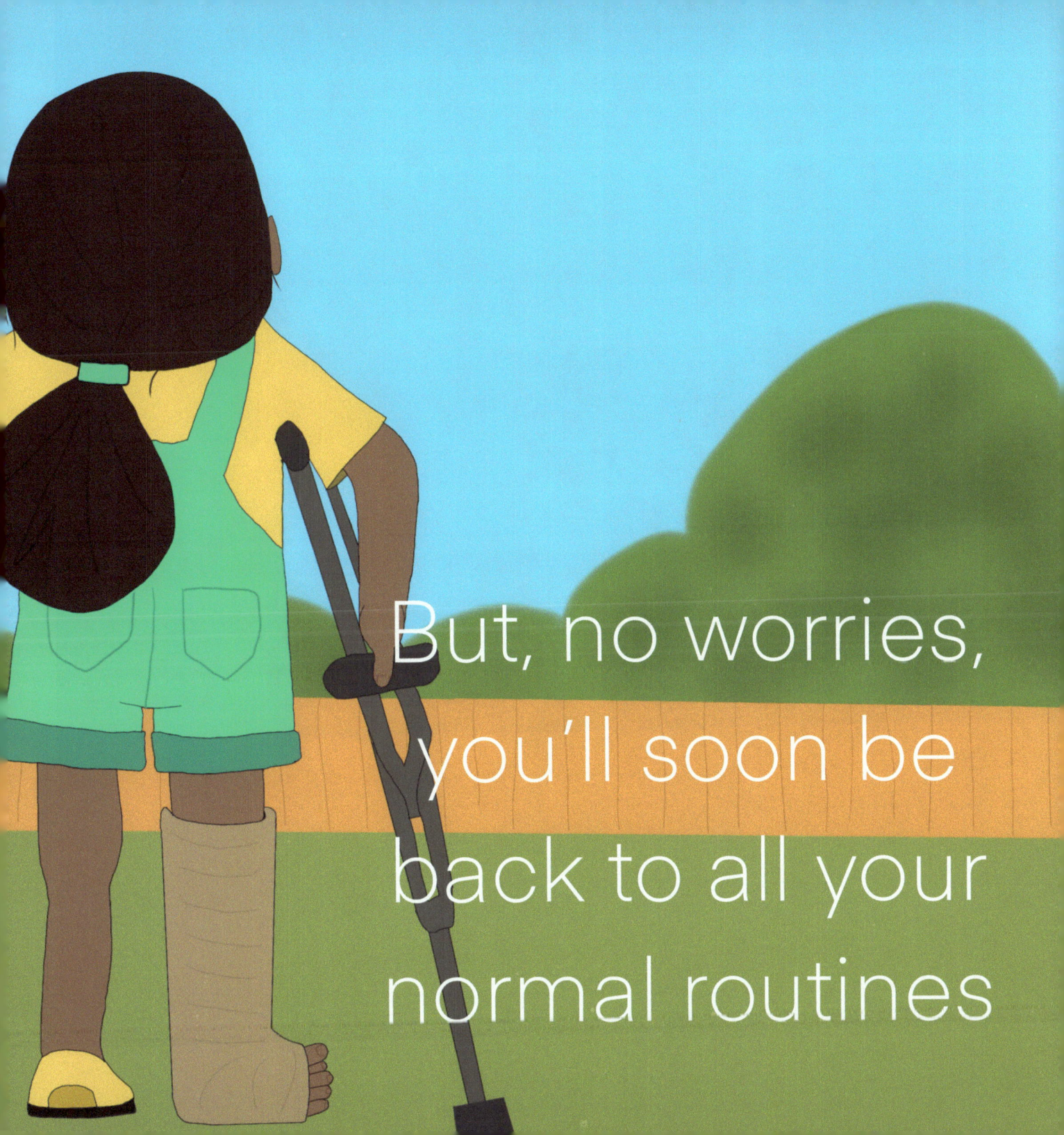

But, no worries, you'll soon be back to all your normal routines

It may get itchy underneath, but never stick something inside

Instead, ask an adult for help. They can blow cool air down the side.

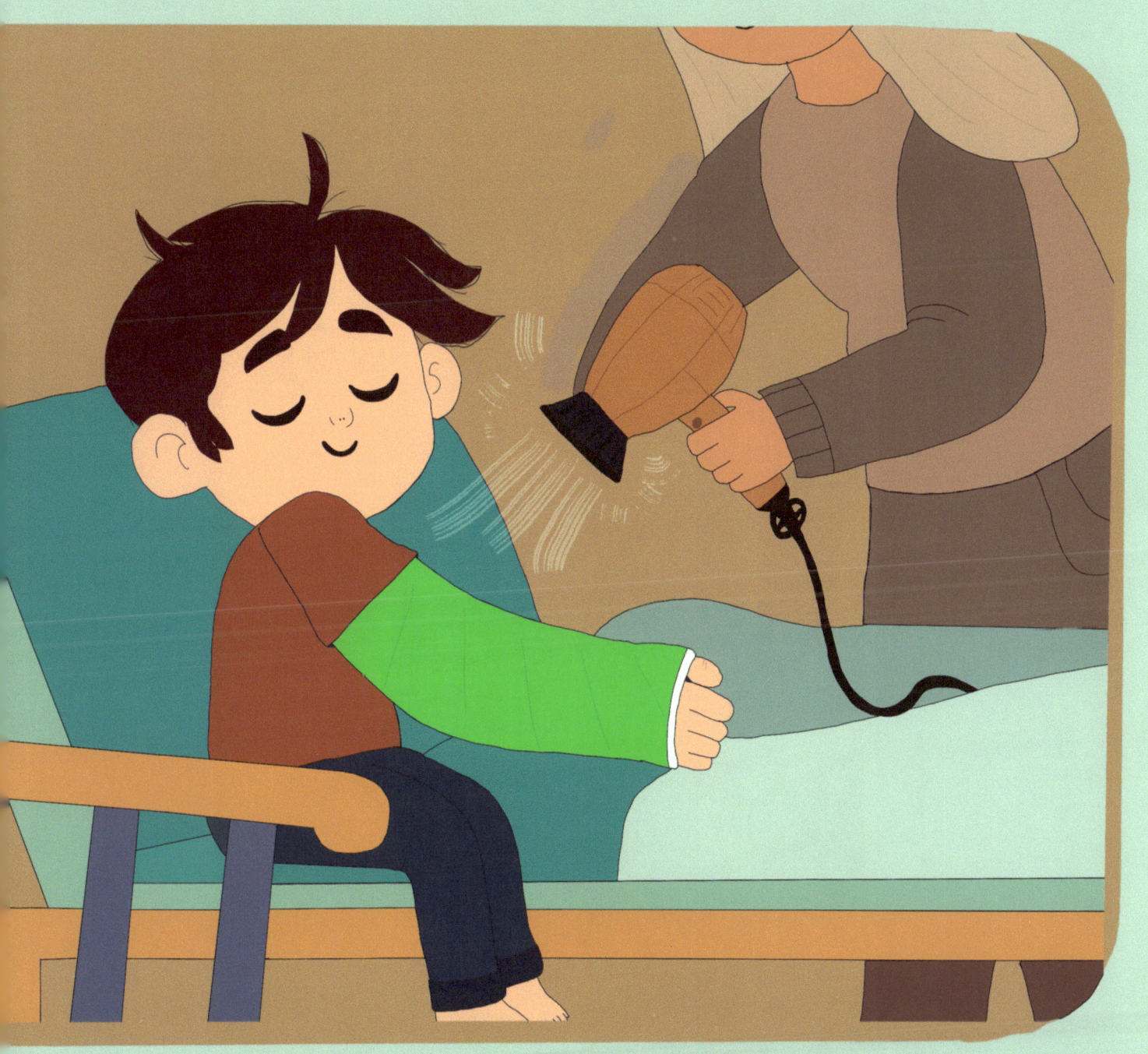

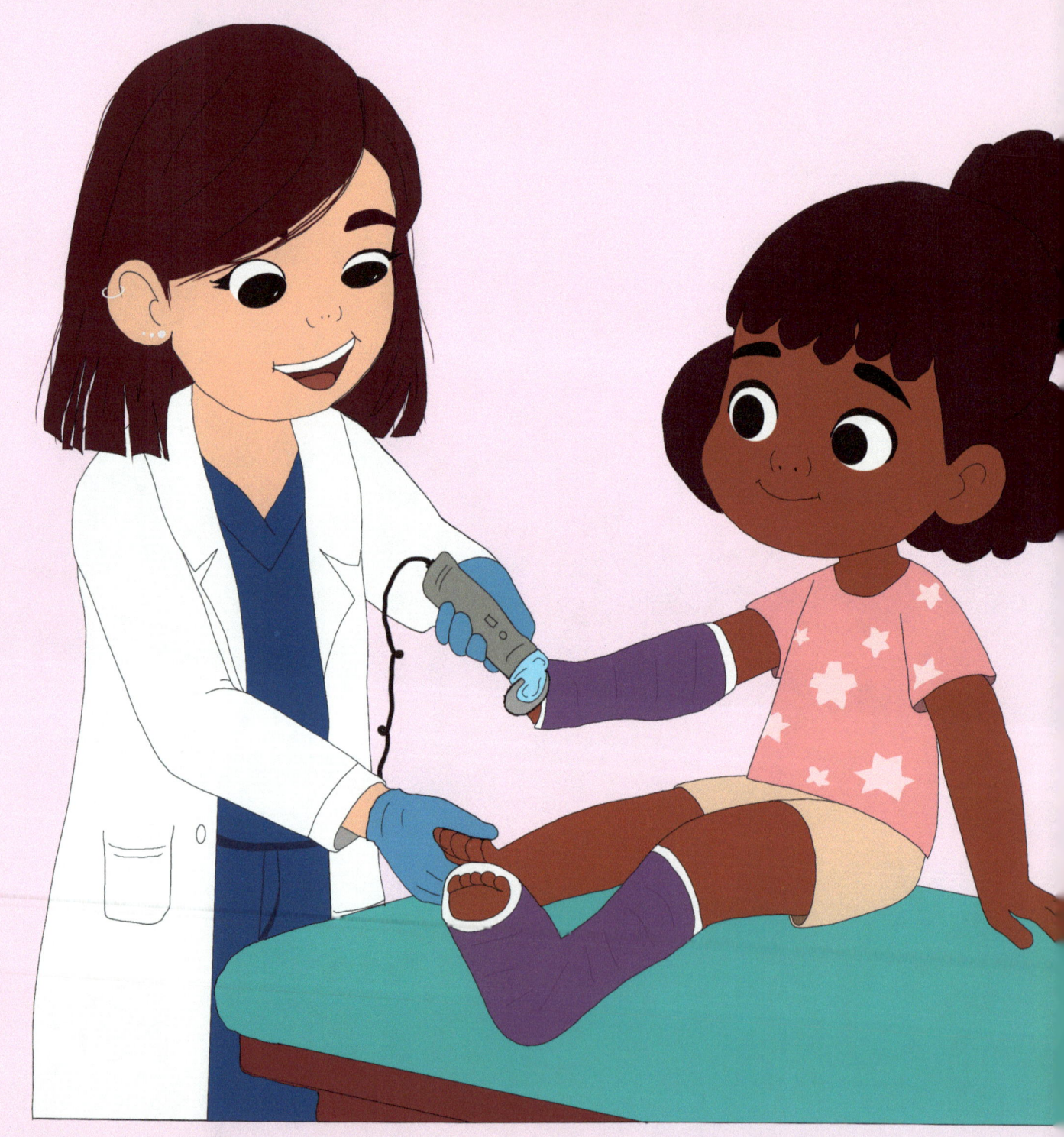

When it's time to take the cast off, the doctor will use a loud tool

It's a safe saw made just for casts —

how cool!

For now we must be patient until your body's hard work is done

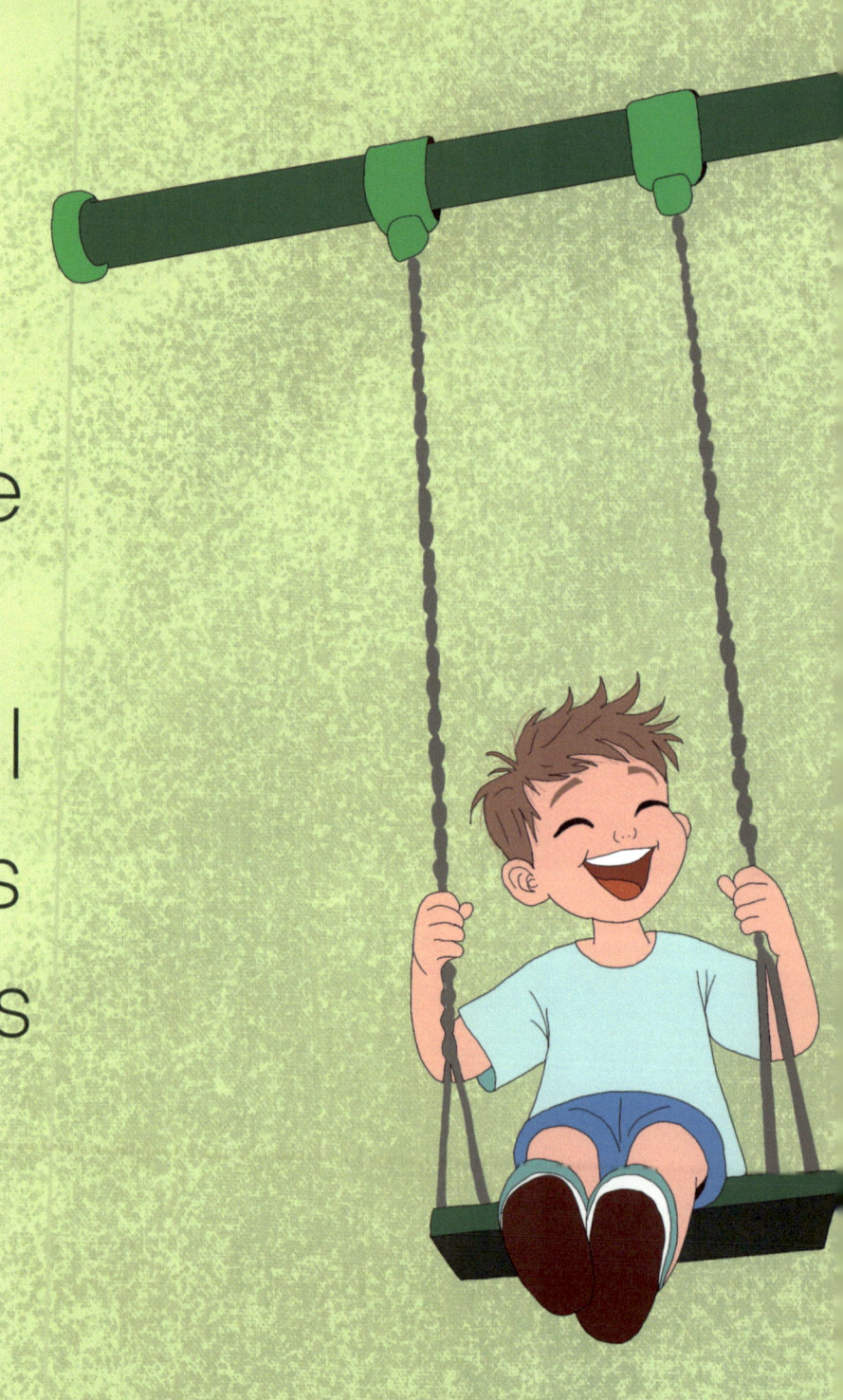

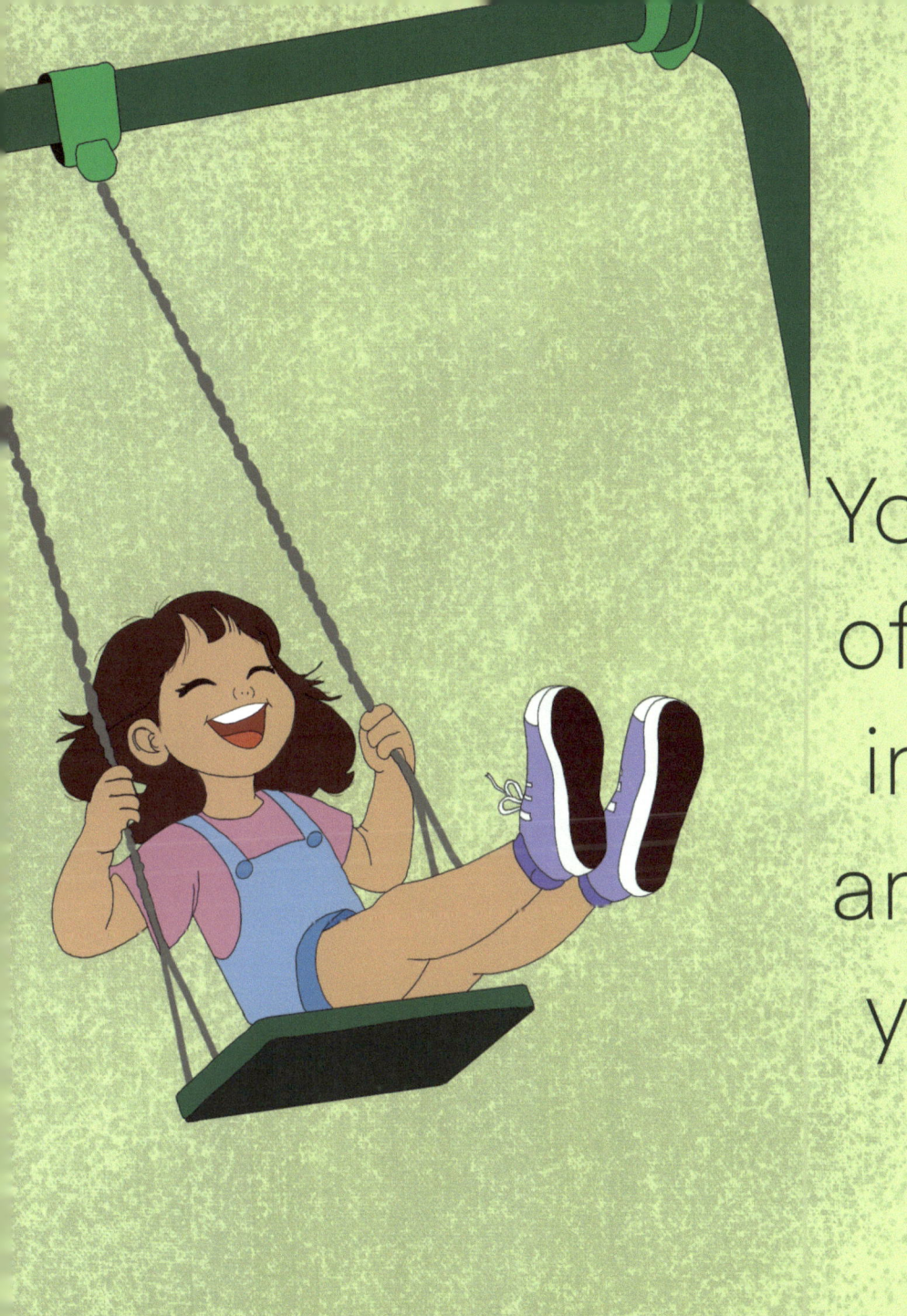

You'll be out
of your cast
in no time,
and back to
your usual
fun

Instructions

If your child's cast gets wet, breaks, or falls off, call the clinic to be seen as soon as possible. If after hours, you should visit the emergency department.

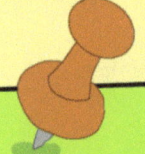

Your child should not participate in sports or gym class or any activities that put them at risk of falling.

Your child should avoid lifting objects with or putting weight on the casted limb

for Parents

It's important to keep the cast dry. Tape a garbage bag around the cast, or use sponge baths.

Watch for any areas of redness or irritation around the cast edges. Pad the edges with cotton or bandaids if it is rubbing on the skin.

My doctor's office:

_____

phone: _____